Milk: A Myth of Civilization

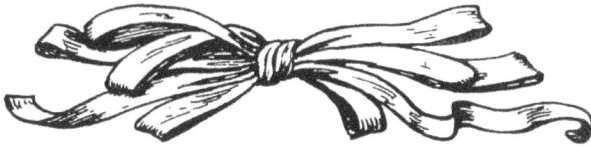

Herman Aihara

George Ohsawa Macrobiotic Foundation
Chico, California

Other books by Herman Aihara include:
Acid and Alkaline
Basic Macrobiotics
Kaleidoscope
Learning from Salmon
Macrobiotics: An Invitation to Health and Happiness with George
   Ohsawa
Natural Healing from Head to Toe with Cornellia Aihara
Rice and the 10-Day Rice Diet with Cornellia Aihara
Soybean Diet with Cornellia Aihara

Contact the publisher at the address below for a complete list of available titles.

This book is made possible through a generous donation from Chris and LisaMarie Nelson.

Keyboarded by Alice Salinero
Text layout and design by Carl Ferré
Cover design by Carl Campbell

| First edition | 1971 |
| Current Printing: edited and reformatted | 2010 Sep 1 |

Published with the help of East West Center for Macrobiotics
   www.eastwestmacrobiotics.com

ISBN -13:978-0-918860-08-8

Contents

Introduction

There was slavery in this country until a hundred years ago. When it was outlawed, another type of slavery was introduced. The new slavery is not black but white. It is not only in the South but all over the country. Armed with intellect, mass media, and science, the new slavery system brainwashed the majority of Americans, including some of the most educated people. This new slavery is the superstition that cow milk is a necessary part of the diet, not only of infants, but of children as well.

The idea that cow milk is a necessary food for humans is a form of slavery, because it is a belief that makes humans dependent on cows. Such a claim is not new. The November, 1959 issue of *Consumer Bulletin* shares this view with me.

"The noted nutritionist who favored more extensive use of milk for 'super-health' expressed the view that milk was the most natural of all nutriments because it is the one thing that nature has evolved for the sole purpose of serving as food. His idea was exceedingly appealing to some prominent dieticians and nutritionists and to workers in agricultural colleges, many of whom were delighted to accept and spread the view that the future health in America was linked to an even greater extension to the parasitism of man upon the cow."

The extension of this parasitism was so great a success that, now, according to the U. S. Government Statistics of 1967, Americans are consuming 80 billion pounds of milk or milk products a year. This consists of 28% of total food consumption and is the highest percentage, followed by meat (20%). In order to meet the demands of such a huge consumption of milk, cows are confined, given hormones and antibiotics and forced to produce milk. This is not only unnatural but also unhealthy.

The U. S. Government frequently gives warning about the dangers of milk in its publication, *Food: Yearbook of Agriculture 1959.*

"An important difference between cow milk formulas and human milk lies in the fact that, while the milk of a healthy mother is always fresh and free from bacteria, any artificial formula must be heat-treated to destroy harmful organisms. Raw milk should never be given to an infant. Even pasteurization cannot be depended on to make milk absolutely safe for young infants."

In other words, cow milk is not only inadequate for human infants (cow milk is for calves only) but is also dangerous. However, milk consumption has increased tremendously within the last fifty years. Why?

The first reason for the increase of milk consumption is that cow milk contains much protein and calcium. Therefore, many nutritionists and dieticians promote the use of cow milk. The second reason is that the dairy industry promoted its consumption through television, radio, and other news media. The third reason is that daily use of cow milk certainly develops man's physical condition. He becomes as fat and as strong as a cow. However, over-use of cow milk deteriorates the human brain to the level of a cow's.

It seems to me that man's happiness depends on his judgment. When his judgment is not man's, he certainly cannot be happy. My aim in writing this article is to encourage man to choose his daily food from the standpoint of man as a part of nature—not from the analytical microscopic theory based on dead life in a test tube. In other words, man should not be a parasite of the cow.

Americans are facing two slavery problems. One is the Negro problem, and the other is the problem of cow milk. Negro slaves were important laborers for the American pioneers who were dependent on slaves then. The cost of this dependence has to be paid. The same thing is true in the case of milk slavery. When man exploits the cow and depends on its milk, he has to pay the cost some day sooner or later, because he who exploits will be exploited.

My Experience with Cow Milk

It was the beginning of October, 1952, when I came to this country, and I was staying with an old farmer in Ohio whom I had known from Japan through correspondence. He had a small farm and raised cows and hens, as well as grew corn. I helped him with milking and gathering eggs every morning. I tasted fresh milk for the first time in my life. It was very delicious and rich.

A month later, I was living in New York City where I couldn't find any milk that tasted similar to what I had had in Ohio. It not only tasted bad, but also caused me to have diarrhea sometimes.

In 1959, George Ohsawa came to this country and gave a series of lectures in 1960 at the Buddhist Academy. Dr. K., one of the attendants, arranged the first macrobiotic summer camp in Long Island, N.Y. Whether or not to use milk was a great concern at the planning of the summer camp, because many young children were expected and milk was believed to be the most important food for the young. Ohsawa emphasized that milk can be used as a pleasure food, but not as a necessary daily food. Thus, milk was eliminated from the camp kitchen. Since then, none of the macrobiotic summer camps have used milk.

We didn't give cow milk to my children until they were about 7 or 8. Then they tasted milk at school or at a friend's home and wanted to drink milk. So we give it to them sometimes. Although they got along without milk, we gave them cheese sandwiches for school lunch sometimes. Giving them milk or milk products once in a while satisfies them, and I don't think this occasional use will harm their physical or mental condition.

History of the Use of Animal Milk

In the Western World

The use of animal milk seems to me to date back to very ancient times. It appears in the Old Testament as well as in the New Testament. According to E. B. Szekely in his *Essene Gospel of John*:

- "Also the milk of everything that moveth and that liveth upon the earth shall be meat for you; even as the green herb have I given unto them, so I give their milk unto you. But flesh, and the blood which quickens it, shall ye not eat." (XXII)
- "Wherefore, prepare and eat all fruits of trees, and all grasses of the fields, and all milk of beasts good for eating." (XXIV)

Many sentences like these appear in the *Bible*. However, there is no evidence that another animal milk was used in feeding a human infant. John H. Tobe asks in *Milk*, "How long would you assume that man has used cow milk to feed infants? If you made the same mistake as I did, you probably believe that man has fed infants cow milk as long as he has used milk as a food or even since his nomadic days when he depended on his herds for what they provided. It came as a shock to me to learn that a man by the name of Underwood was the first to feed cow milk to infants and that was in the year 1793."

Contrary to common belief that the use of milk is ancient, John Tobe claims that cow milk was never drunk by the children in Biblical times after weaning.

In the Western World, the nomadic way of life was the way followed by mankind for thousands of years. And the wandering way of life of these nomadic people may have resulted from the fact that the land was too dry to plant any vegetables. Therefore, instead of harvesting planted vegetables and grains, they learned the art of milking various animals. In order to sustain their life, they had to move constantly where feed was available to their animals. The environmental condition is one of the main reasons that the nomadic way of life was developed. The Bible is the teaching of the way of life that developed among such peoples. Milk was probably an important food for these people and that is why the Bible recommends the use of milk.

In the Eastern World

Contrary to the Western World, the Eastern World didn't rely on much animal milk. This, I assume, comes from the fact that the Eastern people developed agriculture and their life depended on vegetables and grains instead of animal products. The development of agriculture was due to the fact that the land was not as dry and therefore was fit for planting.

According to the *Code of Manu*, the world's oldest human law, which was compiled about two thousand years ago in India and is still the principle law of Hindu, the use of cow milk was prohibited (but not that of the water buffalo). The Chinese and the Japanese rarely used the milk of any animals. However, the use of cow milk was introduced in Japan about 1200 years ago from China, and continued for a short time. A governmental department of milk was even established. However, the use of milk faded away because the environment of Japan did not agree with husbandry, and ill health developed among the milk users. Thus, in ancient times, milk products developed in certain parts of the world where agriculture was difficult. However, in most of the world, people depended on agriculture, which required more intense labor and precision of timing. Because they relied on agriculture, they were able to settle in permanent places instead of adopting the nomadic way of life.

In the Modern World

It is very recently that the use of cow milk became fashionable and almost imperative to the proper growth of children, if not adults. John Tobe wrote in his book, *Milk*, "For approximately fifty years, we have been told that cow milk is the perfect food. Now, who was it that told us or stated the myth that made us believe and accept the fact that milk was the perfect food? I don't know, but believe me, a myth it is. It has no basis in scientific data, fact, experience, or test. Cow milk is not now, and never was, the perfect food for man. In fact, there is loads of evidence available to prove that it is not even a good food, a healthful food, or a suitable food for human beings. The simple, true, unadulterated fact is that milk is a big business and as a big business it is subject to the same sales pitch as any—and that is where the myth of the perfect food and 'drink one to two quarts a day' began."

According to the Statistics of the Department of Agriculture in 1966, Americans consumed foods in the following percentages:

Milk	28%
Animal	20%
Grains	12%
Vegetable	11%
Potato	8%
Fruit	7%
Sugar	7%
Oil	3%
Coffee	1.5%
Ice Cream	1.5%
Others	1%

Human Milk

Life is a miracle. This word is particularly applicable in the case of the birth of a baby and lactation. Milk is a miraculous product of nature. Aspects of it are still unknown—even by 20th century science. The more I investigated the nature of milk, the more questions I had; the answers to which I couldn't find in physiology or nutrition books. For example:

1. When the fetus is in the mother's womb, estrogen and progesterone are supplied in the placenta and help convert the mother's blood to the blood of the fetus. What mechanism controls the secretion of the hormones estrogen and progesterone? How do the hormones convert the mother's blood to fetus blood?

2. As soon as the fetus is born and the placenta separates from the fetus, the secretion of estrogen, progesterone, and lactogen, ceases. Why? How?

3. At the same time, secretion of prolactin from the pituitary gland begins. This "stimulates synthesis of large quantities of fat, lactose, and casein by the mammary glandular cells." (*Medical Physiology* by Guyton) How can this be done? How can the pituitary gland secrete prolactin? What is prolactin? What is the mechanism of milk production in the mammary gland?

4. We assume that mother's milk is a transformation of her blood. A mother may have about five quarts of blood and be producing about three quarts of milk every day. She has to convert more than half of her blood to milk daily. Is this possible? If so, how?

5. Why does the mammary gland produce lactose, instead of glucose (a simple sugar)? (If it produced glucose, its job would be much

simpler because blood has glucose.)

6. If a baby is fed sugar instead of lactose, what will be the effect on the baby's physical condition?

7. If the baby is fed carbohydrates instead of lactose, what will be the effect of this on the baby's physical condition?

One can ask hundreds of such questions.

A Comparison of the Composition of 100 Grams of Blood in a Non-Pregnant Person			
Substance	*Human Plasma	**Human Milk	Change
Water	86	85.2	none
Protein	6-8	1.1	x0.16
Fat	.6	4	x7
Carbohydrates	.6-1	9.5	x10
Ca	.009	.03	x3
P	.003	.01	x3
Fe	.00001	.00001	none
Na	.3	.02	x0.07
K	.02	.05	x2.5
K/Na	.07	2.5	x36
* from *Handbook of Obstetrics and Gynecology*			
**from *Composition of Foods* by the Dept. of Agriculture			

Human milk is usually bluish-white, tastes sweet, and weighs slightly more than water. Essentially, as with all milk, it is an emulsion of fat globules in a fluid. The content of human milk fluctuates from person to person, from birth to birth, and from the start to the finish of the feeding period, whether it is weeks, months, or years. The average composition is 1% to 2% protein, 3% to 5% fat, 6.5% to 10% carbohydrates, and 0.2% salts. The rest is water.

Modern physiology recognizes that milk production does not occur in one day. A mother prepares for lactation throughout pregnancy or even before. According to Guyton's *Medical Physiology,* lactation develops as follows:

1. The breasts begin to develop at puberty. Their development is

stimulated by the hormone estrogen, which is secreted in the monthly menstrual cycle. During pregnancy, tremendous quantities of the hormones estrogen and progesterone are secreted by the placenta. The estrogen and progesterone cause the further growth and development in the breasts that are necessary for nursing. (For specific details of physiologic and anatomic changes that occur, see *Medical Physiology.*)

2. The first fluid secreted by the breasts, colostrum, contains the same amount of protein and lactose as milk but almost no fat. The colostrum is produced in 1/100th the amount of breast milk that will be produced two or three days after the baby's birth.

3. Immediately after the baby is born, there is a marked reduction in estrogen and progesterone, which were formerly secreted by the placenta. Simultaneously, a marked production of the pituitary hormone, prolactin, occurs. The prolactin, formerly inhibited by large amounts of estrogen and progesterone secreted during pregnancy, now stimulates the synthesis of large quantities of fat, lactose, and casein by the mammary gland cells, and the breasts begin to secrete copious quantities of milk instead of colostrum.

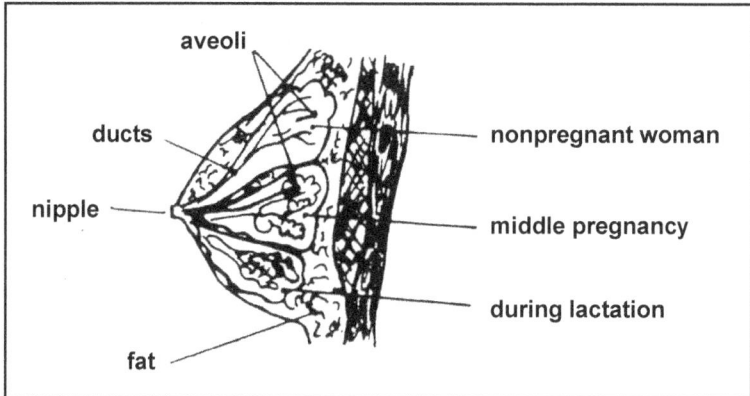

Magnus Pyke gives a good explanation on milk production by the mammary gland in *Man and Food*. "The actual milk-forming cells can more precisely be said to pump glucose (author's note: lactose) and fat through into the milk while holding back much of the protein and some other components, notably sodium and chlorine." See preceding chart.

The process must be a very complicated one because the human mammary gland not only changes glucose to lactose but also the percentages of milk components are quite different from that of mother's blood. As the chart indicates, the comparative amounts in milk versus blood are 10 times more lactose than glucose, 7 times more fat, 3 times more calcium, 2½ times more potassium but less protein (1/7) and sodium (1/15).

In my opinion, and as some physiologists claim, the mammary gland works like a liver or a kidney. I speculate that the mammary gland functions as described below:

Lactose Formation

1. Glucose is delivered to the mammary cells by arterial capillaries.

2. In mammary cells, glucose is converted by insulin (which is yang) to glycogen (which is yangizing because glycogen is insoluble in water). This glycogen is stored in the mammary gland. The liver also converts glucose to glycogen.

3. I suspect that glycogen is formed from certain amino acids, such as alanine, glycine, serine, cystine, and glutamine acid, in blood protein or cell protein. This is the reason the protein in milk is much less than the protein in blood. In humans, it is reduced by 1/7; in cow milk, it is reduced by about 1/2.

4. The stored glycogen is converted to lactose (a double sugar) by prolactin, which is produced in the pituitary gland.

Fat Formation by the Mammary Gland

The mammary gland can store fat supplied from the blood or converted from carbohydrates and protein. Fat deposit starts at puberty and grows greatly during pregnancy.

Mineral Transmutation by the Mammary Gland

Mineral Comparison in Human Milk and Human Plasma			
Minerals	Human Plasma	Human Milk	Changes
Ca	.009	.03	x3
P	.003	.01	x3
Fe	.00001	.00001	none
Na	.3	.02	x0.07
K	.02	.05	x2.5

These changes can be explained by the biological transmutations of the element (see *Biological Transmutation* by Louis Kervran). Sodium will transmute to potassium when combined with oxygen with the help of an enzyme such as lactase.

$$Na^{23} + O^{16} \rightarrow K^{39}$$

This reduces Na and increases K. Some of the K will transmute to calcium when combined with hydrogen, which probably results from the breakdown of water.

$$K^{39} + H^1 \rightarrow Ca^{40}$$

Ca and P are always positively correlated to each other. Therefore, an increase of Ca indicates an increase in P.

The contents of mother's milk change with the growth of the infant, so that mother's milk fits the changing requirements of the infant. In Japan, if the mother does not produce enough milk, she looks for another mother who is nursing a baby of about the same age so that the contents of the milk will be of the right proportions. Such a consideration is rare in modern society where the feeding of cow milk or formula is popular.

Sometimes, it is claimed that the iron content of human milk is too low. However, this is not a shortcoming of human milk (other animals are the same); rather it is an advantage because the newborn baby has plenty of iron stored in his liver or spleen.

In short, mother's milk is best—at least the best available food for an infant. However, it is not the best food for man because it is a secondary product. The mother eats foods, digests them, and produces blood. This blood is converted to milk. Therefore, milk is a secondary food when one considers that vegetables are the first products of nature.

In this sense, any milk is a secondary product—as is meat. In the case of milk, about 7 pounds of protein must be eaten by the mother to produce about 1 pound of protein in milk because the mammary gland changes protein to lactose, reducing its contents 1/7th.

Such secondary food is necessary because infants cannot digest primary foods such as grains and vegetables. Also they can neither assimilate nor regulate the composition because the liver and kidneys are not mature. Milk is in liquid form so it requires neither mastication, which the baby cannot do without teeth, nor long digestion.

Milk can be a perfect food for an infant. However, it is particular food. It is not ordinary food. It should not be served after the teeth grow in for the purpose of mastication. Not many mothers nurse the baby for more than a year. However, modern industry and commercialism promote the use of cow milk after nursing, labeling it a perfect food. This is a mistake from the following point of view:

1. Nutritionally, milk (any) is not a suitable food for children or adults.

2. Using milk as the source of protein is a waste of natural sources. (Nature reduced protein in milk from the blood protein that the parent animal once produced.)

3. Milk reduces the digestive power of the mouth, stomach, and intestines.

4. Milk decreases the transmutation ability, which will lead to an allergic constitution.

5. Brain development is hindered.

6. Milk increases the amount of fat and cholesterol in the body, which may cause high blood pressure or arteriosclerosis.

Cow Milk

Cow milk is produced in the mammary gland of a cow. Compared to cow plasma, cow milk has more glucose (96 times), calcium (12 times), phosphorus (10 times), and potassium (5 times), but less protein (2 times), phospholipids (6 times), and sodium (7 times).

Comparison of Cow Milk to Cow Plasma (from *Man and Food* by Magnus Pyke)			
Substance	**Cow Plasma**	**Cow Milk**	**Changes**
Water	91.0	87.4	x0.96
Glucose	.05	4.8	x96
Protein	7.6	3.4	x0.45
Fat	.06	3.4	x60
Phospholipids	.24	.04	x0.17
Cholesterol esters	.17	trace	total reduction
Calcium	.01	.12	x12
Phosphorus	.01	.1	x10
Potassium	.03	.15	x5
Sodium	.34	.05	x0.15
Chlorine	.35	.11	x0.31

The production of milk in a cow mammary gland must be similar to its production in a human. In other words, functioning as a liver does, the mammary gland converts most of the protein to glucose (but not lactose) and fat.

Mineral transmutation in a cow will also be similar to mineral transmutation in a human. Na changes to K; K changes to Ca, reducing Na and increasing K and Ca. According to Magnus Pyke, "The total amount of milk produced and the proportion of fat in it are affected by the amount of thyroxine (thyroid hormone) circulating in the blood stream of the cow. It has already been suggested that the increase in the butterfat content of milk from cows kept under cold conditions may be due to the increase in the secretion of thyroxine..." This report suggests that thyroxine might be a yin enzyme that promotes the transmutation of protein to fat.

Cow Milk Versus Human Milk

Protein

Cow milk has twice as much protein as human milk and must be diluted before a newborn human can tolerate it. Because it is mostly casein, cow milk forms a large, tough curd when it is mixed with digestive juices. Therefore, the use of cow milk as a food for infants may cause real trouble. Heating cow milk makes curds smaller and softer, but they still tend to curdle in the stomach. Therefore, the infant feels full for about four hours after a feeding. The curd of human milk, on the other hand, is soft and fine. The stomach of the breast-fed baby empties rapidly and easily. Therefore, he wants to eat more often, which, in turn, stimulates his mother's milk production.

The amount of protein in milk, from either a cow or human, is small. However, the proportion of essential amino acids is high. (See *Diet for a Small Planet* by Frances Moore Lappe.) A 5 month old baby will drink 300 ml. of cow milk, which will supply 14 gr. (½ oz.) of protein. However, the same amount of human milk supples only 3 gr. of protein. This is the reason many nutritionists don't consider breast feeding to be good. However, normally the breast-fed baby grows strong and well-balanced. This fact suggests the possibility of the baby having the ability to transmute glucose to protein.

Karen Pryor says in her book *Nursing Your Baby* that "The infant uses the protein in breast milk with nearly 100% efficiency. After the first few days of life, virtually all the protein in breast milk becomes part of the baby; little or none is excreted. The baby fed on cow milk, on the other hand, uses protein with about 50% efficiency, and must waste about half the protein in his diet." This teaches us that too much protein from cow milk may lead to a condition of too little usable protein due to wasting. This fact can be the result of the baby's transmutation—the baby creates or transmutes only necessary components from excess nutrients.

Water

The comment on water in milk by Karen Pryor is excellent. She says,

"Eliminating unusable protein is largely the job of the kidneys. This may place quite a strain on a function that is as yet immature. For years it was widely believed that premature babies gained better on certain formulas than they did on breast milk. Finally, investigators found that the weight gain was due not to growth but to retention of fluid in the tissues. This is the result of strain on the immature kidneys, which are not yet properly equipped to eliminate unsuitable proteins and mineral salts. Human infants get plenty of water for their metabolic needs in their mother's milk. During hot weather, it is the mother who needs extra water, not her breast-fed baby. The baby fed on cow milk, on the other hand, needs water not only for his own metabolism, but to enable his kidneys to eliminate the unusable protein and salts. Thus, he needs water by bottle in addition to the water in his formula, especially in hot weather."

Fat

Fat content in cow milk is about the same as in human milk. (See preceding charts.) However, cow milk contains much more saturated fat than human milk. This is one reason that I am against the use of cow milk after weaning. According to John Tobe in *Milk*, the saturated fat of milk is the first cause of hardening of the arteries (arteriosclerosis).

"Since milk and milk products are saturated fats, their use in the diet must be looked upon as a serious potential source of danger. Its harmfulness has been increased by the even more widespread use of hydrogenated oils in most of our processed foods—and milk or milk products in conjunction with hydrogenated oils make a most 'unholy' and extremely dangerous combination."

"The medical profession for years has been told through the medium of research findings that milk and milk products contribute to the cholesterol build-up in the human body and cause heart attacks. But the profession in general was slow to accept these findings and to pass along this advice to their patients. In fact, many practitioners even today refuse to accept the principle that animal fats are contributors to our causes of heart trouble."

In *Time* magazine, January 3, 1961, an article on the causes of cholesterol and heart disease reports a theory made by Dr. Ancel Keys. It says, "What concerns him much more is the relationship of diet to the nation's No. 1 killer: coronary artery disease, which accounts for more than half of all heart fatalities and kills 500,000 Americans a year—twice the toll from all varieties of cancer, five times the deaths from automobile accidents."

"Cholesterol, the cornerstone of Dr. Keys' theory, is a mysterious yellowish, waxy substance, chemically a crystalline alcohol. Scientists assume that cholesterol (from the Greek 'chole,' meaning bile and 'stereos,' meaning solid) is somehow necessary for the formation of brain cells, given it accounts for about 2% of the brain's total solid weight. They know it is the chief ingredient in gallstones. They suspect it plays a role in the production of adrenal hormones, and they believe it is essential to the transport of fats throughout the circulatory system. But they cannot fully explain the process of its manufacture by the human liver. Although the fatty protein molecules, carried in the blood and partly composed of cholesterol, are water soluble, cholesterol itself is insoluble and cannot be destroyed by the body."

"When cholesterol is deposited in the walls of arteries, Keys says, it is mainly responsible for the arterial blockages that culminate in heart attacks. Explains Keys: As the fatty protein molecules travel in the bloodstream, they are deposited in the intima, or inner wall, of a coronary artery. The proteins and fats are burned off, and the cholesterol is left behind. As cholesterol piles up, it narrows, ir- ritates, and damages the artery, encouraging formation of calcium deposits and slowing circulation. Eventually, one of two things hap- pens. A clot forms at the site, seals off the flow of blood to the heart, and provokes a heart attack. Or, the deposits themselves get so big that they choke off the artery's flow to the point that heart cells die, and the heart is permanently injured."

Dr. Keys' advice for Americans to reduce fat calories in the av- erage U.S. diet by more than one-third, and take an even sharper cut in saturated fats, is to "Eat less fat meat, fewer eggs and dairy products."

This cholesterol theory dealing with atherosclerosis dates back to April 1934 when famous Dr. Timothy Leary, distinguished Boston pathologist, wrote an article called "On the Origin of Atheroscle- rosis" in *Archives of Pathology.* He claimed that arterial changes are produced experimentally in the rabbit by artificial feeding with cholesterol, the amount of which is especially high in eggs, cream, butter, liver, kidneys, milk, and pork. Dr. Leary noted that egg yolk is intended for the embryo and milk for the infant; that "Man is the only animal that ingests eggs and milk throughout its lifetime. Man is also the only animal, as far as is known, that dies in early life from coronary sclerosis, and that acquires atherosclerosis almost univer- sally in advanced life." ("On Milk," *Consumer Bulletin*, November 1959)

Dr. H. M. Sinclair, member of The Royal College of Physicians, teacher of human nutrition at Oxford, noted a lack of unsaturated essential fatty acids (particularly linoleic and arachidonic acids) in cow milk. According to *Consumer Bulletin*, March 1960 issue, "Dr. Sinclair has been cautiously against the overfeeding of children, par- ticularly with cow milk and butter." Excessive use of cow milk and butter (and of margarine of the mass-marketed kind) is one of the causes of essential fatty acid deficiency, which Dr. Sinclair and oth- ers think has an important relationship to the causation of coronary disease, rare in underprivileged countries where milk and butter are not used, and correspondingly common in countries where economic conditions permit these foods to be consumed freely.

Sugar

Breast milk contains about twice as much sugar as whole cow milk. Not only is the quantity of sugar between cow milk and human milk different, but the quality of sugar is different also. The sugar in human milk is largely lactose, whereas that in cow milk includes galactose, glucose, and other compounds.

According to Karen Pryor in *Nursing Your Baby*, lactose is easier for the infant to digest, and its presence makes it easier for the infant to utilize proteins. The author thinks that this fact contributes to the reason that the breast-fed baby eliminates almost no protein. She also reports that a high lactose concentration may help the absorption of calcium.

If sugar is added to raise the glucose content of cow milk, the proper growth of the infant may be severely hindered. In the November 27, 1964 issue of *Time* magazine, a report on infant disease caused by cow milk sugar states that, "When blood and urine tests of infants show an excess of galactose (cow milk sugar), the infant may have trouble in the metabolism of galactose, the symptoms of which are listlessness, failure to gain weight, and jaundice."

"Since the baby cannot metabolize galactose to glucose, the sugar that the body burns for energy, a baby must be put on a special milk-free diet. Otherwise, he is almost certain to develop cataracts, cirrhosis of the liver and, if he does not die, to be mentally retarded."

Why use cow milk and risk such danger and expense?

Lactobacilli in Milk (from *Fundamentals of Bacteriology* by Martin Frobisher, Jr.)

"The organisms of this germ are widely distributed in soil, on plants and around barnyards, and are frequently present in market milk,... although possibly not in such large numbers. They are important in the dairy industry in several ways. Lactobacilli, as their name implies, are associated with lactic acid production."

"While commonly found in milk and cheese (they are important in the ripening of cheese), certain species are also found in large numbers in the intestinal contents of infants (L. bifidus) and in the vagina (L. acidophilus), while others occur in souring vegetable products like ensilage and sauerkraut. They are rarely associated with disease but a few cases of infection due to them have been reported. They grow well in milk at a temperature of from 300 to 600 C."

"In certain countries lactobacilli have been used for hundreds of years in combination with certain yeasts and streptococci to produce beverages of fermented milk. The yoghurt (L. bulgaricus) of eastern and central Europe, the busa of Turkestan, the kefir of the Cossacks, the koumiss of Central Asia, and the leben of Egypt are examples of these."

"In this country, Lactobacillus acidophilus is used to produce a similar fermented milk product called 'acidophilus milk'."

"Metchnicoff observed that, among people drinking these sour milk beverages, longevity was common. He attributed this to the beneficial effects of the soured milk, and particularly to Lactobacillus bulgaricus or the 'Bulgarian bacillus' found in yoghurt and leben. He became the foremost exponent of the idea that if these fermentative organisms could be implanted in the intestine, life might be prolonged. This is probably erroneous."

"It was found later that L. bulgaricus cannot grow in fluids having low surface tensions, while L. acidophilus, a closely related species, can. Bile produces low surface tension, and it may be due to this that L. bulgaricus cannot be implanted in the intestine, since the intestinal contents contain bile."

John H. Tobe says in *Milk*, "Elie Metchnicoff, the famed Russian biologist who was director of the Pasteur Institute and winner of the Nobel Prize in physiology and medicine in 1908 (along with Paul Ehrlich), laid down the principle that the human body can protect itself to a great extent against the invasion of unfriendly bacteria by its own resources. He observed that in the human intestines a diverse flora of both friendly and unfriendly organisms exist and that the presence of the friendly colonic organisms implanted into the infant's digestive tract with the first few drops of the breast milk is a vital development of nature and is also most essential for the later years. This was the principle of his famous theory of phagocytosis."

"It has been provided by nature that breast milk contains a group of complex intestinal bacteria flora vitally important in establishing normal conditions in the intestinal tract of the infant. It is called Lactobacillus, and it is invariably found in high concentration in breast milk."

"This intestinal bacterial flora, once implanted in the infant, should by normal continuance and multiplication last a human being till the end of his days."

"It is my contention that this intestinal bacterial flora will protect a human being against most allergies. I further suggest that the widespread affliction of allergies is mainly due to the lack of, or too weak or inefficient, intestinal bacterial flora."

"There is no reason to doubt that this intestinal bacterial flora can be acquired from various live enzyme-containing foods over a period of time. But an infant, child, and adult would have a much better chance of health if these organisms were supplied at birth, as nature intended and provided for."

"Typhoid fever, mumps, scarlet fever, and measles are seldom if ever contracted by nursing infants. Therefore, it is believed that human milk gives immunity from certain diseases."

"One important contribution of human milk sugar," according to *Nursing Your Baby*, "is its effects on the bacteria that grow in the baby's intestines. The process of digesting lactose creates an acid medium in the baby's intestinal tract, whereas other sugars result in an alkaline medium. Many bacteria cannot survive in an acid medium. The intestinal tract of the artificially-fed baby, on the other hand, with its alkaline contents, supports the growth of many organisms, including harmful and putrefactive bacteria. That is why the stool of the artificially-fed baby has the usual fecal stench, while the stool of the breast-fed baby has no unpleasant odor. The intestinal contents of the breast-fed baby are practically a pure culture of one beneficial organism, Lactobacillus bifidus. By-products of bifidus metabolism make the infant's intestinal tract even more resistant to the growth of other, invading organisms."

It continues: "Dr. Paul Gyorgy, discoverer of Vitamin B_6 and pioneering researcher into human milk and nutrition, found that human milk contains a sugary compound, the bifidus factor, which is not found in the milk of cows, and which is essential for the growth of many varieties of L. bifidus. The bifidus factor and the acid medium resulting from the digestion of lactose in breast milk promote the establishment of a safe and protective bacteria in the newborn and, thus, offer him real protection against invading organisms."

Also bottling or other means of feeding may cause oxidation of milk and growth of undesirable bacteria. Therefore, breast feeding can be recommended because milk is drunk from breast to mouth without being exposed to the air.

Dr. Keiichi Morishita, one of the first physiologists to claim that blood is made in the intestine from food under normal conditions, wrote about milk in the macrobiotic magazine in Tokyo. My translation appears in the following several chapters.

Lactobacilli (by Dr. Keiichi Morishita, author of *Hidden Truth of Cancer*)

There are about 100 types of lactobacilli known today. Two or three kinds, however, are most important for humans:
1. Lactobacillus bulgaricus
2. Lactobacillus acidophilus
3. Lactobacillus bifidus.

Lactobacillus bulgaricus exists in raw cheese. Lactobacillus acidophilus has a strong resistance to acid and is a main component of the lactobacilli beverages. Lactobacillus bifidus is present in infants who are nursed by their mother's milk. The properties of these lactobacilli indicate their extreme importance for our health:
1. They decompose sugar and produce lactic acid.
2. They have resistance to acid. This is especially true of the lactobacillus acidophilus, which resists stomach acid and is able to

reach the intestine.

3. They produce vitamins, but we can produce them if we have these bacilli in our intestines. However, if we eat much meat and sugar, a bacteria called anoilinase grows in the intestines and destroys these vitamins. Thus, it is of no use to eat foods that are rich in vitamins when we have the anoilinase bacteria in our intestine. With respect to the nutrition of food, we must consider not only its composition but also its physiological change in our body.

4. They produce a growth factor that enables children to develop.

5. Lactobacilli are good for the prevention of food poisoning. Oysters often cause poisoning, but if one has lactobacilli in his body, he can prevent this reaction. Typhoid fever, dysentery, and cholera are not solely caused by their bacteria, as is believed by current medical theory, but actually are caused more by lack of lactobacilli in our intestine. If we have enough lactobacilli, we will not be affected even if we ingest some cholera bacteria.

These important lactobacilli decrease proportionally with aging. This tendency is greater among meat-eaters. Vegetarians can live longer because the lactobacilli in their intestine decreases less with aging. The idea of drinking milk to supplement the lactobacilli, lacking in the meat-eating Western countries, may seem plausible. However, present pasteurized milk has no value at all in this respect.

A baby who has been nursed by its mother has many lactobacilli bifidus. However, when the baby is fed artificially, these bacilli disappear and, instead, various unimportant bacilli grow. Such a baby acquires a weak constitution with body cells that are not sound.

By changing to breast milk after feeding a baby with artificial food, the lactobacilli will increase. The reverse is also true. The food value of milk exists only when lactobacilli are present. This bacilli is important for the proper growth of children. In nature, a baby drinks only breast milk directly from its mother's breast. If, however, the milk is extracted from the breast, heated to the boiling point and then given to the baby, the baby will not grow. If this continues, the baby will soon die. The reason for this is that the lactobacilli have been destroyed by the high temperature of heating.

Pasteurization of milk involves two processes:

1. Low heat (140°F) sterilization. This process is aimed at killing the chloroform organism which, according to scientists, is harmful to humans. This process, however, also sometimes kills the important and useful lactobacilli.

2. Addition of preservatives. The preservatives used in pasteurized milk also have a destructive effect upon the lactobacilli of milk. Even if lactobacilli are added with the preservatives, pasteurized milk is no longer milk. Even a baby cannot grow from it. Several years ago, the U.S. Dept. of Agriculture experimented by feeding calves pasteurized milk. These calves died within three months.

Pasteurized milk is a poor milk because it not only lacks lactobacilli, but also contains preservatives which may kill our own lactobacilli. If pasteurized milk has any value at all for us, it is that of a bowel loosener. Since pasteurized milk has preservatives and a protein which differs from our own, the intestines rejects it. The result is a condition of diarrhea. By nature, human babies do not like cow milk. Usually, they will refuse it. However, if a baby likes cow milk, it should be a warning that the baby's constitution is somewhat similar to that of a cow.

In addition, if a person's health is improved by drinking milk, it indicates that his constitution is also similar to that of a cow's. It is somewhere between that of a human and a cow. These conditions, of course, are a result of the mother's drinking a lot of milk during pregnancy. Thus, the baby was adapted to cow milk at birth.

People today eat many poisonous foods such as meat, canned foods, processed foods, dyed foods, etc. Then, the drinking of milk acts as a laxative or cleaner. Therefore, they are unknowingly cleansing their systems by drinking much milk. However, taken from this standpoint, the calcium and nutritional value of milk is meaningless because it does not stay in our body.

Pasteurization

Pasteurization, according to *Funk & Wagnell's Encyclopedia*, is the process of heating a liquid, particularly milk, to a temperature between 131°F and 158°F to destroy harmful bacteria without materially changing its composition, flavor, or nutritive value. If this definition of pasteurization is right, there is no real pasteurization in the market because all pasteurized milk is changed in flavor, nutritive value, and composition by heating. The process was named after the French chemist, Louis Pasteur. He created the process that bears his name purely to save the wine-makers in France from going bankrupt. (See *Macrobiotic Monthly*, Vol. 9, No. 6.) Due to uncleanliness and other factors, the wine was turning sour before it could be sold and something had to be done about it. So Louis Pasteur found a way of killing off the germs or bacteria that were causing the trouble. In this way, he saved the wine industry. However, he had nothing to do with the pasteurization of milk.

The pasteurization of milk is a gimmick created by commercialism—money-making greediness under the names of sanitation and life saver. It is a fact that the dairy business is a large one and it would probably never have grown to its present proportions if pasteurization had not gone into effect. Pasteurization definitely makes milk last longer and makes its handling easier. Also, because of this, it is possible to use milk in a great variety of products.

Milk and milk products make up 28% of the weight of food Americans eat. The dairy products hold the largest share of the American farmers income.

Contrary to its original intention or definition of pasteurization, it destroys much, if not most, of the value contained in milk. As Dr. Morishita claims, pasteurization kills important bacteria. Also, most of the vitamins are destroyed. Most vegetarians do not rely on milk as a vitamin supply. However, people who eat much sugar need lots of vitamins. Therefore, the lack of vitamins in milk will bring trouble in handling sugars.

"It was found that the pasteurization and normal handling of milk alters vitamins C, E, K, B_1, and Riboflavin. It also alters the enzyme growth factors and anti-stiffness factors. Protein and calcium molecules are changed as well."

"One of the strongest arguments in favor of pasteurization is that it prevents us from falling victim to disease spread by dirt and filth. In my opinion, this amounts to nothing else but buck-passing. It is a suggestion that we cannot trust our farmers and our dairymen. It is a suggestion that our Dept. of Agriculture and our Health Dept. are unable to guarantee us clean, wholesome milk." (*Milk* by John Tobe)

It is very strange that most nutrition authorities of today advise people not to cook because of the destruction of vitamins and enzymes. Yet, they say that milk should be pasteurized. This contradiction does not make sense. In any case, whole raw or unpasteurized milk contains all the known vitamins in proportions corresponding almost completely to the requirements of the animal body. Pasteurization will destroy this. However, I will not argue this point further because I do not recommend cow milk for human consumption anyway.

Vitamins

Cow milk contains only 1/2 to 1/10th the essential vitamins contained in human milk. This is interesting because a cow eats mostly raw grasses, which supposedly contain a lot of vitamins. On the other hand, a human mother eats mostly cooked foods, if she is not a raw vegetarian, and yet her milk contains far more vitamins. Is this an indication that cooking destroys vitamins but will help us produce our own vitamins? This is the major reason why formula-fed infants must have vitamin supplements or some food supplements. Breast-fed babies, on the other hand, do not need any outside source of food until around the age of five or six months. Even then, breast milk continues to be a good source of the vitamins they need.

Breast milk contains plenty of the fat-soluble vitamins A and E. "At the age of one week, the breast-fed newborn has more than five times the amount of vitamin E in his system than does the bottle-fed baby," says Karen Pryor.

Vitamin D controls the baby's ability to absorb calcium. The fat-soluble vitamin D does not normally come from diet except in northern and Arctic climates. In the rest of the world, vitamin D is synthesized in the body upon exposure to sunlight. If the baby does not receive enough sunlight, he may have rickets due to the failure to absorb Ca. However, the breast-fed baby is unlikely to develop rickets until he is weaned.

The Sept. 1965 issue of Time magazine reports a case of vitamin D abuse: "One pregnant woman in Baltimore, who was eating well, drinking a great deal of milk, and taking her prescribed multivitamin capsules, was getting 2,000 to 3,000 units of vitamin D daily along with her sunshine, as against a recommended daily intake of only 400 units, even for a fast growing child. Such overdoses of vitamin D sometimes cause unnatural calcium deposition in the fetus; its bones, especially the base of the skull, grow unusually dense, and chalky deposits narrow the aorta. Sometimes it causes mental retardation."

Interestingly enough, vitamin C is contained in large quantities in breast milk but it is almost completely absent in even unpasteurized cow milk. From a macrobiotic point of view, I suggest that a cow can produce vitamin C by itself from its food. When a cow converts blood to milk in the mammary gland, vitamin C and vitamin B convert to a more yang substance, probably to protein, because a cow's mammary gland is located in a very yang position (the lowest part of the cow's body). On the other hand, the human mammary gland is located in a fairly yin position; therefore, it can convert blood to a fairly yin substance. As a result, human milk contains a lot of vitamin C. Production of vitamin C through the human mammary gland is so effective that scurvy, the disease caused by a deficiency of vitamin C, has never been seen in a breast-fed baby, even in the case where the mother has scurvy.

Calcium in Milk (by Dr. Keiichi Morishita)

"The abundance of Ca in milk is another reason the modern theories of nutrition recommend drinking milk. The calcium theory concerning human health goes roughly as follows:

"The existence of a healthy condition is due to the abundance of Na and Ca in our system. In the event of an increased level of K and Mg compared to Na and Ca, sickness will follow. Therefore, we have to eat foods which contain substantial amounts of Na and Ca."

I agree that our blood must have abundant Na and Ca because from my experience a healthy blood contains more Na and Ca than unhealthy blood. However, I do not agree in recommending milk to obtain Ca.

Na and Ca are elements that come mainly from animal foods. K and Mg are elements that come mainly from vegetable foods.

According to the Kervran-Ohsawa Transmutation Theory, these four elements can transmute each to the other. Ca can be made from Mg, which is present in chlorophyll, by the addition of oxygen.

$$Ca_{20}^{40} \leftarrow Mg_{12}^{24} + O_8^{18}$$

From this it is possible that we can have enough Ca when we eat only vegetables. (Translator's note: Moreover, a cow eats just grasses and yet has a large bone structure.)

A baby calf weighs about 130 pounds when born. He will weigh about 240 pounds one month later. By this time, he is already walking around. This rapid growth rate requires quick development in body structure; in other words, bone growth in order to meet the need required by activity and weight. This is the reason cow milk contains so much calcium—it contains 3-4 times that of human milk.

On the other hand, human milk contains phosphorus. This element is very important for brain growth and development. The human baby develops its brain first, while the animal develops its bone structure first. Therefore, milk for a human and for that of an animal naturally should be different. Giving cow milk to the human infant, without thinking about such an order of nature, is too simple-minded.

The present scientific analysis lacks precision when it states cow milk is the same and as good as human milk. Science measures calories, vitamins, proteins, sugars, etc. However, they do not know exactly how cow milk makes cows and human milk makes humans. For example, what kind of elements in milk cause the formation of a cow's horn?

When science reaches a more complete understanding of the difference between cows and humans, it will declare that cow milk should not be given to humans.

Cow milk is for a calf. When it is given to a baby, he will grow rapidly (physically) as does the calf. However, the mentality does not grow and develop. Our constitution and mentality is a result of what we eat. Therefore, we must depend on the right food for humans ... not for cows.

In most parts of the world, enough of the vitamin B complex is supplied to breast-fed babies by their mothers whatever the diet, except in the case of southern Asiatics where mothers eat only white rice. However, not all the vitamin B needs may be supplied by cow milk, especially when it is pasteurized.

Iron

Many nutritionists worry about the low content of iron in human milk. However, cow milk, in fact, contains less iron than human milk does. Furthermore, the amount of iron in human milk is the same as the amount in the mother's plasma. Therefore, this should not be considered as a small amount. According to Karen Pryor in *Nursing Your Baby*, "The baby is born with a good store of iron in its liver, and with a high concentration of red blood cells, which is presumably diluted to normal over a period of growth. If the mother is not anemic during pregnancy, the baby's stores of iron are probably adequate for the first year of life, even on an exclusively milk diet."

This is understandable from the macrobiotic viewpoint because a baby is very yang, as the result of nine months of feeding on its mother's blood. Therefore, iron-rich foods, such as egg yolks, will cause too yang a reaction in the baby, even in the case of cow milk feeding. (U.S. Government Food recommends egg yolks to three month old babies as a source of iron.)

Allergy to Milk

Time magazine, in the October 1966 issue, reported that, "Countless peptic-ulcer patients are put on a bland diet rich in milk and cream. If they then get cramping abdominal pains, nausea and diarrhea, even worse than their original complaints, their doctors usually put them on a still blander diet—meaning more milk. If such patients shirk their milk drinking and their symptoms diminish, the usual explanation is a quick, glib suggestion that they must be allergic to milk. Not so, reported two University of Colorado doctors in the *Journal of the A.M.A.* The trouble is far more likely to be a shortage of the enzyme that the body uses to digest milk (lactase). For such patients, more milk means only more trouble."

"To use lactose as fuel, the body must first break it down into two simpler sugars: glucose and galactose. The enzyme that does the cracking is lactase. Nature intended babies to live on milk, and lactase deficiency is fortunately a rarity in the newborn, but the incidence increases with advancing age"

An article from the *New York Times* called "Doctors Warn of Intolerance to Milk" reports, "The bulk of the world's non-white adult population is probably intolerant to milk, studies by United States and Australian scientists, released yesterday, indicated. The scientists said that their findings raised serious questions about the advisability of shipping powdered milk to nutritionally deprived persons in Africa and Asia."

"They said that although non-white children seemed to be able to digest milk, intolerance often started to develop during adolescence and became well-established by adulthood."

"In a report published in the current issue of the Journal Science, Drs. Shi-shung Huang and Theodore M. Bayless of John Hopkins University Medical School said that milk intolerance was apparently due to the lack of an enzyme, lactase."

"The enzyme is needed to digest the milk sugar, lactose. Lactase is produced by the lining of the small intestine."

"The consequences of milk intolerance vary somewhat from person to person, but they usually include abdominal bloating, cramps, and diarrhea after drinking more than a glass of milk, the doctors reported. In the studies at the Baltimore University, 19 of 20 healthy Oriental adults, living in the United States, were intolerant to milk and lactose."

"An earlier study by John Hopkins scientists indicated that about

70 percent of adult American Negroes were unable to digest milk. A similar percentage of milk-intolerant persons was found among African Negroes in Uganda."

"Bayless said that he hoped the findings of a high percentage of milk intolerance among non-white adults would be a warning to doctors who prescribed large quantities of milk to pregnant women and ulcer patients."

Doctors say that those people are intolerant to cow milk. However, from the standpoint of macrobiotics, those who are intolerant to milk are probably healthier than those who have no trouble drinking milk. An adult's condition is not fit for milk drinking, especially another species' milk. Scientists, as a result of their analytical studies, have forgotten the more basic principle of life.

When Mother's Milk Is Not Enough

If for some reason she does not have enough milk, a mother should eat mochi or drink koi-koku (carp soup) or miso soup with mochi.

Rice Flour Mochi Recipe

> 5 cups sweet brown rice (pressure cooked)
> 7 cups sweet brown rice flour
> 5 cups water

Rinse rice in pan of water until water becomes clear. Soak 24 hours. Put soaked rice in pressure cooker, cover and cook using a flame a little higher than medium. Bring to full pressure, turn down and cook for 20 minutes. Turn off and let stand for 45 minutes. Mix flour with very hot rice and pound with a Surikogi (wooden pestle). Wet both hands in cold water and knead rice. Dip hands in cold water each time to handle hot rice. When all rice grains are broken down, the kneading process is completed.

Bring water to boil in a steamer pan. Put a wet cloth inside pan after it begins to steam. Place raw mochi on top of the wet cloth and cover with the same cloth. Cook at a high heat for 20 minutes. Pierce mochi with a dry chopstick. If nothing sticks to it when it is withdrawn, mochi is done. Select a mochi and dip it in the covering you prefer. If you make 3 inch flat, round shaped mochi, cover with 1 teaspoon cooked aduki beans to make Daifuku (mochi stuffed with cooked red beans).

Coverings

1. Sesame Mochi: Roast and grind black sesame seeds. Add pinch of salt and boiled water. Mix until creamy and cool. Dip cooked mochi in sesame seeds. Coat on all sides.

2. Nori Maki Mochi: Bake one side of Nori over flame. Cut in 6 pieces. Dip mochi in soy sauce and wrap with Nori.

3. Walnut Mochi: Roast walnuts lightly and grind strongly until oil comes out. Add pinch of salt or soy sauce and a few drops of boiling water. Mix until creamy and cool. Spread on cooked mochi.

Azuki Mochi

> 1 cup azuki beans
> ¾ cup water
> 1 tsp salt
> ¼ cup 'yinnie' syrup (barley-rice syrup)

Soak azuki beans overnight in 2 cups of water. Bring to boil in regular cooking pan. Add ¼ cup cold water and bring to boil again. Repeat this process 4 more times with ¼ cup cold water. Cook until beans are tender. Add ¼ cup 'yinnie' syrup. Cook 20 minutes, then add salt and cook 10 minutes more without a cover until the excess liquid has cooked off. Let cool. (Azuki beans are yang; pressure cooking may make them taste bitter.) Cover hot, soft mochi with azuki beans.

Kenchin Zoni (Mochi with soup)

> 1 daikon (4") cut in large chunks, then chunks cut in
>   1/3" sections each section cut in 1/16" rectangular
>   slices
> 1 carrot (4") cut in pencil shaving slices
> 1 burdock root (6") cut in pencil shaving slices
> 5 taro (albi or sato imo) cut in thin rounds
> 1 scallion cut in 1/3" rounds
> 1 Tbsp oil
> 1 Tbsp soy sauce
> 1 tsp salt
> 7 cups water

Saute burdock until smell is gone. Add daikon, taro, a pinch of salt, and carrot and saute for 10-15 minutes. Add water and cook for 30 minutes. Add rest of salt, soy sauce, and scallions. Turn off heat. Drop in mochi and bring to a boil. Serve with minced nori crumbled on top of soup.

Carp Soup (Koi-koku)

> 1 carp
> 3 times as much burdock as carp
> 3 heaping Tbsp of miso soybean paste
> 1 Tbsp oil (optional)

Tie into a bag or cheese cloth green tea leaves that have been used for tea. Remove the bitter part of the carp (gall bladder) carefully so that it will not burst. Do not remove the scales. Cut up the fish into half inch pieces. Shred burdock and place in pot with carp. Put the bag of used tea leaves on top. Add enough water to cover. Cook 3 hours or until the bones are soft. Take out tea leaves. Dilute miso soybean paste with a little water and pour over the carp. Cook for an additional hour. The mother should eat everything in this dish including the bones, so that she can get plenty of calcium.

Wakame Miso Soup with Mochi

> 5 cups boiling water
> 1 large handful wakame
> 1/3 cup bonita flakes or fish powder (optional)
> 1 Tbsp miso soybean paste
> 2-3 pieces mochi

Soak wakame 10-15 minutes. Wash well. Chop and add to boiling water. Season with bonita flakes. Cook 20 minutes, add miso and mochi, and stir well. Cook about 10 minutes more and serve.

Milk Substitutes

Western medicine recommends fruits and much vegetable and animal protein in order to increase the quantity of milk. However, excess fruits or vegetables may produce more milk, but it will be thin, watery, and not nutritious. Such milk may result in an anemic child.

If the mother still does not have enough milk, the ideal substitute for mother's milk is special rice cream or kokkoh.

Special Rice Cream

> 1 cup brown rice
> 10 cups water
> ¼ tsp salt

Wash rice and toast in a dry pan, stirring constantly until golden and the rice begins to pop. Add water and salt then cook for about 2 hours or more on a low flame. Squeeze out the cream with a cheese cloth or cotton cloth.

Milk: A Myth of Civilization

Kokkoh Feeding Chart

Age	Kokkoh/Water	Times per Day	Quantity per Feeding	Quantity per Day	Calories
1 day	1½ tsp - ¾ c	0-2	1½ T	0-3 T	—
2 days	1½ tsp - ¾ c	3-5	1 T	3-5 T	6
3 days	1½ tsp - ¾ c	5-6	2 T	10-12 T	15
4 days	1½ tsp - ¾ c	7	3 T	1c 5T	30
5 days	1½ tsp - ¾ c	7	5 T	2c 3T	50
6 days	1½ tsp - ¾ c	7	6 T	2c 10T	120
7 days	1½ tsp - ¾ c	7	7 T	3c 1T	140
2 weeks	1 T - ¾ c	7	8 T	3½ c	320
4 weeks	1 T - ¾ c	7	8 T	3½ c	320
2 months	2 T - ¾ c	6	11 T	4c 2T	380
3 months	2 T - ¾ c	6	14 T	5c 4T	450
4-6 months	2 T - ¾ c	5	18 T	5c 10T	520
7-8 months	2 T - ¾ c	5	20 T	6c 4T	570
9-12 months	2 T - ¾ c	5	20 T	6c 4T	570

Kokkoh No. 1

> 35% brown rice
> 60% sweet brown rice
> 5% white sesame seeds

Kokkoh No. 2

> 55% brown rice
> 25% sweet brown rice
> 5% white sesame seeds
> 15% oatmeal

All ingredients are first roasted, then mixed, and ground up to a fine powder. (A stone grinder is best but a blender is all right.) For approximate feeding of kokkoh, see the chart on page 40.

For cooking kokkoh, use 1½ teaspoons with ¾ cup water at the first one week feeding. From the second week to one month, use 1 tablespoon with ¾ cup + water. From the second month, use 2 tablespoons with ¾ cup water. Mix well.

The feeding chart is an approximation. If the baby wants more than the amount shown in this chart, he can have more. As the baby approaches teething period, he should be given rice that is first chewed by the mother. (This is not necessary with kokkoh, however.)

Conclusion

I will quote various books because so many words have been stated by wise men on milk, I find no reason to use my own words. Jack Dunn Trop, the president of Natural Hygiene Society, wrote in *You Don't Have to be Sick!*: "Modern science is so wonderful that a mother doesn't have to nurse her baby anymore. Most honest, well-informed pediatricians will admit that there is no substitute food for a child that can compare with its own mother's milk. Mothers have stepped off their pedestal. A baby's mother is now Bessie the Cow. Although the cow is a docile, contented, placid, dumb animal, no member of the bovine family is as stupid as the mother who thinks that cow milk can nourish her baby as nature intended. Cow milk is best for a calf but not for a human baby."

Arnold Ehret said in *Mucusless Diet Healing System* that milk: "...also makes a good glue for painting. Cow milk is too rich for adults and for babies, and plainly destructive. A baby's stomach cannot digest what a calf can. If milk must be used, then add at least half water and some lactose. Cottage cheese with stewed fruit is good for a transition diet. All other kinds of cheese are highly acid and are mucus formers."

Otto Carque in *Vital Facts About Foods* has excellent views on milk. He said, "Milk and milk products are far from being absolute necessities for the maintenance of the health and vigor of the race. The milking of animals is an unnatural process. It lowers their vitality and often makes them victims of disease, while it impairs the quality of the milk. Milk and dairy products are by no means staple foods with all people. The use of milk is comparatively recent in origin in the history of the human race, and even today there are people like the Japanese who hardly take any milk."

Karen Pryor in *Nursing Your Baby* states: "As far as infant nutrition goes, all we can say with complete certainty is that breast milk is the only completely adequate food for the first six months, and forms a splendid addition to the diet thereafter. In a reasonably healthy mother, breast milk has all the needed nutrients."

I will finish my article with George Ohsawa's writing, which is taken from his book, *Jack and Mitie*. (The English version is to be published in the near future by the George Ohsawa Macrobiotic Foundation.) "In India there are as many cows as there are in all the European countries put together. They are extraordinarily respected like mothers. Yet, the people do not drink much milk as the statistics (one person per thousand Europeans drink milk) would indicate. In reality, there are hundreds of millions of people who do not drink it once in their lives. All the more, they do not kill the cow. It is considered the mother of the nation and symbol of the god of love and goodness. In Maiden Park in Calcutta, which is one of the biggest parks in the world, there are always hundreds of cows walking around. It is a real park with cows. They stroll along the streets and if a cow happens to sit down on the great boulevard, the tramway, bus, or any traffic stop, everyone waits until it removes itself. One cannot hit a cow. They are respected and beloved mothers of the nation. They are free."

"Here in the West, the cow has the right to live only on the condition that it gives its milk, its meat, its blood, its gelatine, and its skin. It lives to be exploited and killed. It looks at man as the most cruel animal in the world."

"Here, in the West, one drinks milk. In Paris alone, they drink millions of quarts per day. In England, one estimates the annual consumption of milk and dairy products at $25 million; in the United States, several times this amount. More than 80% of the whole agricultural product of England is of animal origin, economically speaking."

"In the West, one exploits the animals or depends for his existence on them. The cell of bone and flesh in the Westerner is constituted mostly of animal food."

"One drinks milk and eats animal meat. What is most lamentable is feeding nursing babies and children cow milk. Western women have abandoned the maternal qualifications. They are deprived of the glory of being a mother. By taking cow milk, their babies become brothers and sisters to the calf. Man's children become adopted by animals. No animal makes its offspring a milk-brother and sister to other animals. Even the Romans did not make their children into calves."

"In the countries of the Far East, one considers the embryological and lactation periods as the most important for the psychological formation. Following next in importance is the physiological formation, which depends fundamentally on the nutrition of the first period. The foundation of all existence rests in the creative eating we do during our first years."

"Why does one make his own child a suckling to the animals? The primitive man does not understand at all."

"It is Western medicine that recommends milk as the best nutrition for the baby. Why? Because animal milk is nearest to human milk in chemical composition. But, what logic is this! Here is another superstition like that of fruit and meat. The son of man is not the son of animals. He cannot and should not be. The son of man is the son of man and nothing else."

"Don't we realize the distinct intellectual, moral, sentimental, spiritual, aesthetical, linguistic, sensorial, and social differences between a calf and the son of man? How do we identify a calf with the son of man? How incredible!"

"It is here that we can and must find the origin of all Western misconceptions of the constitution of the universe, including superstition and ridicule to which the mentality of the 'civilized' clings tenaciously."

"East is East, West is West..."

"That is why force is the supreme law in countries of the 'civilized,' just as in the world of carnivorous animals."

My intention in compiling this book is to try to clarify the misunderstanding that cow milk is a perfect food for human consumption—by infants and children as well as adults. I am not against the use of milk for one's pleasure on occasion. The use of milk or milk products for pleasure and to make one's life amusing and joyous would be an interesting subject. Such a subject will be discussed in some cookbooks.

Modern civilization is perverted in its direction, as ample evidence shows. One of the most important causes of such perversion, in my opinion, lies in man's eating habits. Because one third of the total consumption of food in this country consists of cow milk, Americans must give serious consideration to whether or not cow milk is good food for man.

Appendix

About Milk Products and Chemical Additives

A friend of mine, who hadn't had any fish or meat for four years, experimented by eating 2 ounces of Monterey Jack cheese every day. He had to stop the experiment after only 5 days because the rash that developed on his skin was very itchy and started to bleed.

This cheese was bought at a respected natural health foods store in San Francisco. The rash was gone in 3 days after stopping the experiment.

He had a much sharper reaction to cheese than most Americans, because his kidneys were not used to handling animal protein and the toxins that cheese might produce.

However, if such toxins stay in our tissues, the result will be worse. For instance, a chronic stiffness of the tissue might develop from the unsaturated fat of the cheese. Also, excess Ca in milk and cheese may cause kidney stones and gall bladder stones.

Such toxins are not serious when compared with toxins from regular supermarket milk products. Here is a list of chemicals that are contained in some milk products:

1. Lucerne Processed Cheddar Cheese
   ascorbic acid added as a preservative
2. Lucerne Cream Topping
   dextrose
   sorbitan monostearate
   artificial flavor
   carrageenan
   propellent gases: nitrous oxide
   chloropenta-flouroethane

3. Modillac—a liquid infant formula for nursing bottles
    skim milk
    water
    dextrin-maltose-dextrose (derived from corn)
    corn oil
    mono and diglycerides
    calcium
    carrageenan
    sodium ascorbate
    niacinamide
    tocopherol acetate
    vitamin A palmitate
    calciferol
    thiamin
    hydrochloride
    pyridoxine phydrochloride

4. Carnation Instant Breakfast (chocolate malt flavor)
    sucrose
    malted milk
    sodium caseinate
    lactose
    corn syrup solids
    monocalcium phosphate
    artificial flavors
    sodium silic aluminate
    ammonium carrageenan
    sodium ascorbate
    ferric orthophosphate
    vitamin A
    niacinamide
    riboflavin
    thiamin
    mononitrate
    basic copper carbonate
    pyridoxin hydrochloride

The recently published book *Get Your Health Together* by Joan Weiner has a good report on food additives and chemicals.

"Antibiotics are fed to milk cattle, and poultry are dipped into antibiotic baths in order to prolong their shelf life when marketed."

"Heavy tranquilizers are given to cows so they won't panic while riding to the slaughterhouse."

"Diethylstilbesterol, or simply stilbesterol, is mixed with cattle feed to make them gain weight fast."

"Strontium 90 is found in milk."

"Diacetyl, a chemical scent, is used to prevent loss of buttery smell when butter is stored."

"Hydrogen peroxide, for bleaching, and magnesium oxide, for neutralizing, are used in butter."

"Ice cream flavors sometimes contain ethyl acetate (pineapple, for example), a plastic solvent whose vapor is irritating to mucous membrane; piperonal (vanilla) also used to kill lice; butyraldehyde (nut) used in rubber cement and synthetic rubber, aniline dyes and plastics."

Bibliography

1. Carque, Otto, *Vital Facts About Foods*, Natural Brands, Inc., Los Angeles, CA, 1940.

2. Ehret, Arnold, *Mucusless Diet Healing System*, Ehret Literature Publishing Co., CA, 1953. (A good article on milk.)

3. *Food: the Yearbook of Agriculture 1959*, The U.S. Government Printing Office, 1959. (An authoritative book on nutrition. There are many valuable informative facts on not only milk but also other foods and on law, cost, etc. Worthwhile to read.)

4. Guyton, Arthur C., *Textbook of Medical Physiology*, W. B. Saunders Company, Philadelphia, PA, 1971.

5. Lappe, Frances Moore, *Diet for a Small Planet*, Ballantine Books, Inc., New York, NY, 1971. (Her advice on protein is very interesting. She recommends fish and dairy products as sources of protein.)

6. Norris, P. E., *About Milk, Cheese and Eggs*, Thorsons Publishers, Ltd, London, 1972.

7. *Prevention*, February, 1971, "Milk is not For Grown-ups."

8. *Prevention*, April, 1971. (On the chemicals that are contained in creamed cottage cheese selling in the U.S. markets.)

9. *Prevention*, August, 1971. "Poor Countries Won't Thank Us for Milk"

10. Pryor, Karen, *Nursing Your Baby*, Harper & Row, New York, 1963. (Very clear writing. The best book on milk; there are also other excellent articles about breast feeding, delivery of the baby, etc.)

11. Pyke, Magnus, *Man and Food*, McGraw Hill Co., New York, NY, 1970. (General information on milk.)

12. Szekely, Edmond B., *Essene Gospel of John*, Shambala Pub-

lications, Inc., Berkeley, CA, 1968. (Advice on diet by the Essenes.)

13. Tobe, John H., *Milk*, Modern Publications Reg'd, Canada, 1963. (Strong argument against the use of milk.)

14. Trop, Jack Dunn, *You Don't Have To Be Sick!*, Natural Hygiene Press, Inc., Chicago, Ill., 1961. (Highly philosophical book on diet.)

About the Author

Mr. Herman Aihara was the founder of the George Ohsawa Macrobiotic Foundation, the sole purpose of which is the education of macrobiotics in the Western world. He worked on macrobiotic education in the United States since he was elected the first president of the Ohsawa Foundation in New York City in 1960. His lecturing covered many cities including the San Francisco Bay area, Los Angeles, Seattle, and Portland once a week or once a month. However, his biggest tours were for summer lectures that covered the entire country, followed by many summer camps.

He edited many publications of G.O.M.F. such as *Macrobiotic*, a monthly magazine, and *Macroguides*. His book, *Macrobiotics: An Invitation to Health and Happiness*, was a great success, and is still considered by many as one of the best books for people just beginning a macrobiotic diet.

About Dr. Keiichi Morishita

Dr. Morishita, an extraordinary medical doctor, was one of the few scientists who confirmed that blood is made in the intestine by food under normal physical conditions.

He was a unique man in medicine who was interested not only in his specialty but also in philosophy, astronomy, and in the macroscopic origins of life.

Dr. Morishita was an unusual individual who lived what he believes. Although he ranked high in the eyes of the medical fraternity, he was a practicing macrobiotic.

Majoring in blood physiology, he took his undergraduate work at Tokyo Medical University, graduating in 1930. In 1935, he received his doctor of medicine degree and was later appointed Assistant Professor of Physiology at Tokyo Medical University. He taught at the Dental School of the University in 1937 and in 1944 became the Technical Chief for the Tokyo Red Cross Blood Center. He also was a member of the Physiology Association of Japan, President of the Life Sciences Association, and Vice President of the New Blood Association.

The author of many research papers for the academic community, Dr. Morishita wrote many books for the layman and general public. They include:

The Origin of the Blood Cell
Foundations of Physiology
The Degeneration of Life
Blood and Cancer
Hidden Truth and Cancer

Hidden Truth and Cancer was translated and published by the George Ohsawa Macrobiotic Foundation (Macroguide No. 2).

A list of books by George Ohsawa and others on macrobiotics can be obtained from the George Ohsawa Macrobiotic Foundation, PO Box 3998, Chico, CA 95927-3998; 530-566-9765; fax 530-566-9768; *gomf@earthlink.net.* Or, visit *www.ohsawamacrobiotics.com.*

www.ingramcontent.com/pod-product-compliance
Lightning Source LLC
Chambersburg PA
CBHW022134280326
41933CB00007B/685